Leabharlann na Rinne
Ringsend Library
01-2228499 1|2|22

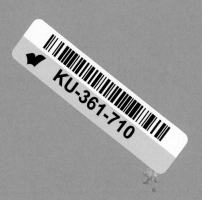

KU-361-710

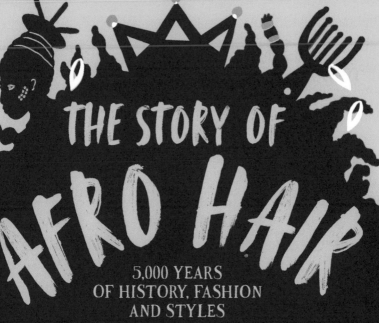

THE STORY OF
AFRO HAIR

5,000 YEARS OF HISTORY, FASHION AND STYLES

WRITTEN BY
K.N. CHIMBIRI

ILLUSTRATED BY
JOELLE AVELINO

■SCHOLASTIC

Acknowledgements: Thanks to Sandra Gittens for sharing her knowledge of Afro hair type. I would like to express my deepest gratitude to Sally-Ann Ashton, Darren Chetty, Debora Heard, Avril Nanton, Jy'Mir Starks, Danny Thompson, Robin Walker and Tony Warner for taking time out of their busy schedules to offer constructive feedback on parts of the text. I'd also like to thank Stephen Bourne for his help with specific queries. Thanks also to my agent, Julia Churchill, for making this possible and Leah James at Scholastic for her wonderful editorial support.

Finally, I'd like to thank all my friends and family for their huge support and patience with this project, in particular: Mum, Dad, Amanda, Angel, Dee, Diana, Mia and Rosemary.

Published in the UK by Scholastic, 2021
Euston House, 24 Eversholt Street, London, NW1 1DB
Scholastic Ireland, 89E Lagan Road, Dublin Industrial Estate, Glasnevin, Dublin, D11 HP5F

SCHOLASTIC and associated logos are trademarks
and/or registered trademarks of Scholastic Inc.

Text © K.N. Chimbiri, 2021
Illustration © Joelle Avelino, 2021

The right of K.N. Chimbiri and Joelle Avelino to be identified as the author and illustrator of this work has been asserted by them under the Copyright, Designs and Patents Act 1988.

ISBN 978 07023 0741 6

A CIP catalogue record for this book is available from the British Library.

All rights reserved.

This book is sold subject to the condition that it shall not, by way of trade or otherwise, be lent, hired out or otherwise circulated in any form of binding or cover other than that in which it is published. No part of this publication may be reproduced, stored in a retrieval system, or transmitted in any form or by any other means (electronic, mechanical, photocopying, recording or otherwise) without prior written permission of Scholastic Limited.

Printed in Italy by L.E.G.O.

Papers used by Scholastic Children's Books are made from wood grown in sustainable forests.

2 4 6 8 10 9 7 5 3 1

www.scholastic.co.uk

* The map in this book is for illustrative purposes only and should not be relied on for accuracy.

CONTENTS

INTRODUCTION:
WHAT HAIR STYLE TO WEAR?

For most of history, people throughout the world, who lived in the same area tended to wear their hair in the same way as those around them. It was like this in ancient Africa too.

Hairstyles showed which group someone belonged to. They could also show a person's position in their group. Leaders and rich nobles' hairstyles were often fancier than everyone else's to show they were more important.

Sometimes people choose to wear their hair in a style because they like it, however, that doesn't mean the style is fashionable! The hairstyles which society considers in fashion at any moment in history are decided by hair type, climate, culture and religion. Sometimes hair fashions are started by **trendsetters** (like rulers, celebrities and famous hairdressers).

In the past, Africans wore hairstyles that were very different from European hairstyles. Not only did they have different hair types but the cultures,

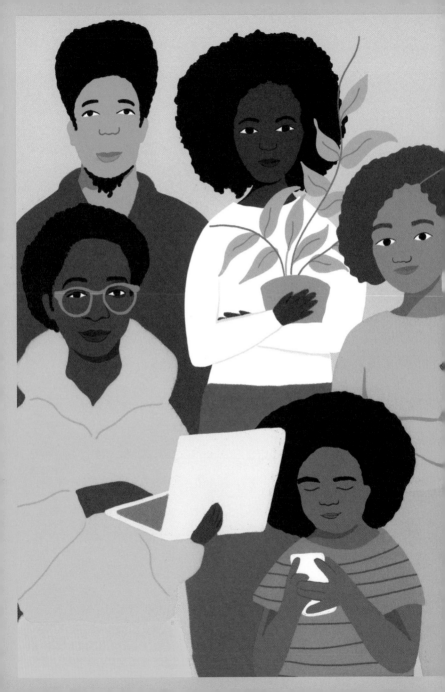

religion, climate and leaders on their continents were different. Later on, although the hair type was still the same, when other things changed (like culture, religion and leaders), the hairstyles people of African descent considered fashionable slowly changed too. This book will tell you about a few of the styles people have worn throughout history.

CHAPTER ONE:
WHAT IS AFRO HAIR TYPE?

Hair starts with the skin. Each strand of hair grows out of a pocket in the skin called a **follicle**. Hair grows all over the body (usually it doesn't grow on the palms of the hands, soles of the feet, lips and a few other areas). The hair on our bodies is short, the hair on our heads is longer than body hair. Most of the hair on our heads grows out of the scalp. Most men, and some women, can grow the hair on their face into beards and moustaches.

Hair type is partly decided by the follicles. The shape of the follicle helps to shape the hair as it grows out of the skin. The follicle shapes the hair to make it coily, curly, wavy or straight.

People with Afro hair type have curved hair follicles. As the hair grows out of the curved follicle, it curls and twists into a coily shape. Some people have very coily hair shapes; others have much looser coils. The way the coily hair grows out of the curved follicles helps to make Afro hair grow up and out rather than downwards like other hair types.

Hair is mostly made up of a protein called **keratin**. Keratin is the same material that our nails are made of. The way the keratin is distributed inside every strand of hair also helps to make the hair coily. Afro hair type doesn't have keratin spread evenly along the inside of each hair strand.

A gland attached to the hair follicle produces an oil called **sebum**. Sebum travels out of the scalp and

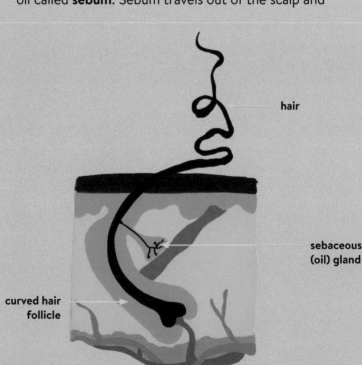

hair

sebaceous (oil) gland

curved hair follicle

along each strand of hair like a car on a road. If the road is straight the car can just zip along the road. However, if the road is bendy, the car must travel much slower and sometimes the bends in the road force it to stop altogether.

So, Afro hair tends to be drier compared to other hair types because it's much more coily and the oil cannot travel up the hair easily.

Afro hair is very delicate. All the twists, curls, bends and coils in every strand of hair are a point of weakness. So, if the hair is combed or brushed too hard it can break or be easily damaged.

All this gives Afro hair its unique **textures**. So, although Afro hair needs to be handled gently, it's so versatile and can be fashioned into many different hairstyles. For thousands of years, it's been worn in a wide variety of ways. Some styles showed messages. Others were worn just for fashion or fun. But all these hairstyles make up the story of Afro hair.

CHAPTER TWO: ANCIENT AFRICAN HAIR STYLES

ncient Egypt is the most famous ancient African kingdom. The ancient Egyptians wore a wide variety of hairstyles. Many of their hairstyles from more than 5,000 years ago are very similar to those which people with Afro hair wear today. They wore locks, plaits (sometimes with **extensions** to make the hair look longer), twists, wigs, short natural cuts and longer loose, curly hair.

Elite men and women wore expensive wigs. At first the wigs were short and simple but over thousands of years the wig styles got bigger and fancier! Some wigs even had *hundreds* of long plaits.

Although their hair was often short, women did want to grow their hair longer. One ancient Egyptian recipe uses the fruit and oil from the castor-oil plant to help the hair to grow.

Children usually had all their hair shaved off except for

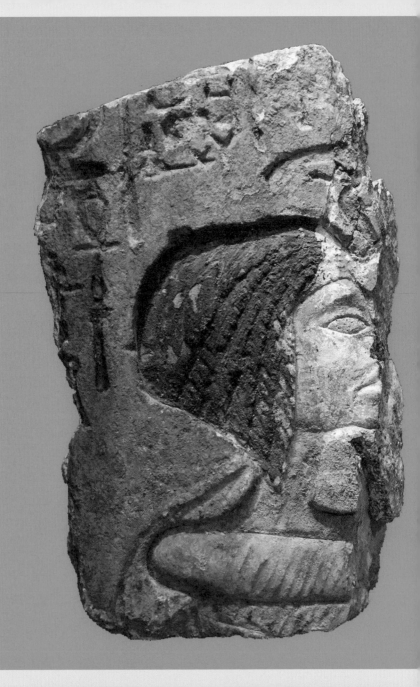

one thick plait on the right-hand side of their head. Sometimes children wore styles with parts of the head shaved and parts with hair.

A famous queen called Nefertiti often wore this hairstyle. Many **Egyptologists** call it the 'Nubian wig'. However, no one really knows for sure if this was a wig or was Nefertiti's own hair worn in the style. The style was first worn by soldiers in the Egyptian army who came from the Sudan. After Nefertiti wore the style, wealthy ancient Egyptian men and women copied it.

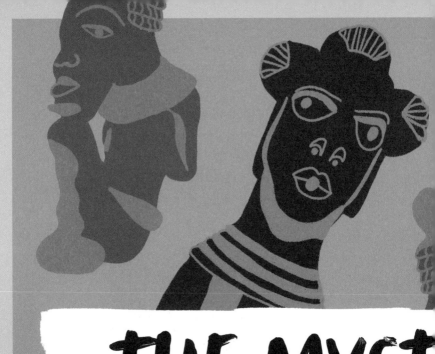

THE MYST

Meanwhile, more than 3,000 years ago in West Africa (today's Nigeria) there was an ancient civilization called Nok. The ancient Nok civilization is thousands of years old, but its beginnings and history are a total mystery to us today. All that

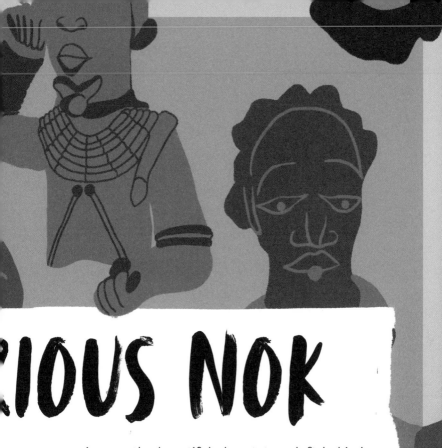

IOUS NOK

remains are the beautiful clay statues left behind by the ancient Nok people. Many of these statues show men and women wearing fancy hairstyles that must have taken hours to create.

CHAPTER THREE: MEDIEVAL AFRICA

reat Benin was a kingdom in West Africa. It was located in the south of today's Nigeria. Great Benin was ruled by kings called *Obas*. The *Oba* lived in a huge palace. Inside the *Oba*'s palace were some rooms decorated with beautiful brass plaques. These sheets of brass showed important events from Benin's history. Today, we call these plaques the Benin Bronzes.

The Benin Bronzes show us a wide variety of hairstyles, which were important, as they showed the wearer's position in society. The photo on the next page shows one of the Benin Bronzes. This man's hair and beard told everyone that he was an **Olokun** priest. His hair is worn in even-sized **locks** with three plaits or twists. He also wears three feathers from a special bird in his hair.

In the 1400s, Europeans began coming to West Africa to trade. Over the centuries they often described the hairstyles they saw. One Portuguese traveller who visited Africa in the 1400s wrote that

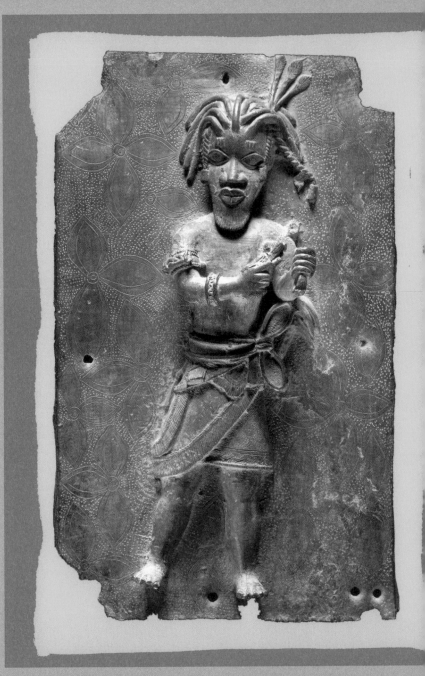

the hair he saw was short and was 'weaved and tied' ('weaved' meant 'plaited') into neat styles.

Another European writing hundreds of years later noticed that people took good care of their hair. It was worn 'in an hundred different Fashions'. He also wrote that as well as using wooden and ivory combs, which they carried around in their hair, the hair was dressed with palm oil and charcoal 'to keep it black and make it grow'. Then, it was decorated with 'gold toys or pretty shells'. Some people, he said, wore styles with part of the hair shaved off. And the writer mentioned that 'They are fond of their Beards and comb them daily...'.

Most people with Afro hair lived in Africa but as well as Europeans visiting Africa, some Africans also came to Europe, including Britain. During early Tudor times, fashionable white

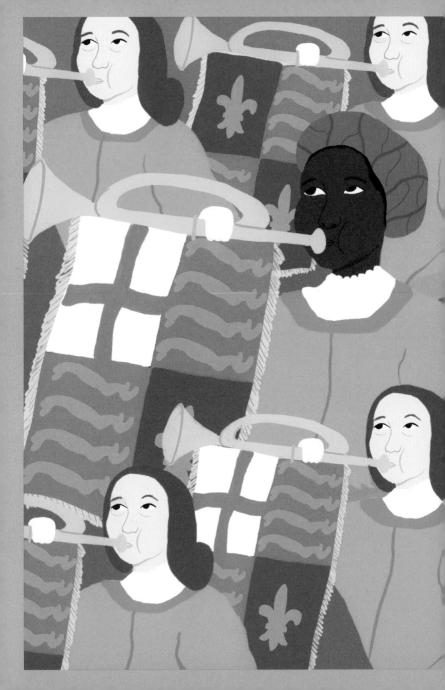

English men wore long hair. King Henry VIII wore his hair long at first too.

John Blanke was a Black musician who worked for Henry VII and Henry VIII. We can only see a bit of his hair in this picture, the rest is covered. His clothes are exactly the same as the other trumpeters, who are white, and his face is **clean shaven** too.

Later on in Henry VIII's reign, when the French king, Francis I, cut his hair short after a knock to his head, Henry VIII copied his style. From then on, he liked to wear his hair short and grow his beard.

In the 1600s, France became the leader of European fashion in clothes and hairstyles. Soon England, and later, America watched France to see the latest fashions in hairstyles (as well as clothes). And soon hairstyles from France would begin to influence people with Afro hair too.

CHAPTER FOUR: EUROPEANS COLONIZE THE WORLD

(1500 TO 1899)

uropean nations began to compete with each other to build up **empires**. At first the Portuguese and the Spanish had the biggest empires. Later on, other European countries like the Netherlands, England, France and Denmark–Norway began claiming **colonies** to build up their empires. Soon England, later Britain, became the main world power. Millions of Africans were taken, against their will, by Europeans to the colonies in North, South and Central America and the Caribbean as enslaved workers.

The enslaved people had to work very hard. They were forced by slavers to work without pay. They had no freedom and were treated poorly by their enslavers. The enslavers had the law on their side. Most enslaved workers toiled for Europeans and people of European descent in mines, forests or on plantations (big farms) that grew crops like sugar, tobacco, cotton or rice. A very small number of enslaved men and women worked as domestics

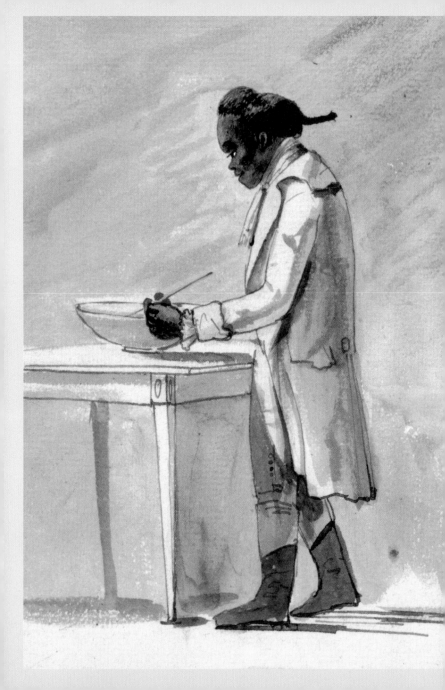

or personal servants. This means they did physically less demanding work than in the fields, mines or forests. They worked in the house carrying out tasks like cooking, cleaning and looking after their owners and their family.

Some of the personal servants were skilled hair stylists and barbers. Some were enslaved men and women who learnt how to style European hair and take care of wigs. Others were enslaved men who knew how to shave their owners' beards and make and look after their wigs. Sometimes the enslaved African men who worked in the slaver's house were made to wear wigs themselves. These wigs were made from European hair. At the time poorer Europeans, usually women, often sold their hair to earn money. It was then used to make wigs for wealthier white people, especially white men. Wearing a human hair wig showed wealth and a high position in society, especially for men.

BRITAIN'S COLONIES IN THE AMERICAS

Britain's slavery mostly took place in its Caribbean colonies. However, the slave owners often came home to Britain. Then, they sometimes brought their enslaved personal servants with them. It became a **status symbol** to own enslaved African servants.

Most enslaved people weren't brought to Britain though. They remained in the colonies in North America and in the Caribbean. They had to work such long hours that they did not have much free time to recreate the fancy hairstyles they had worn in Africa. During their free time the enslaved workers had to fit in many tasks like looking after their own little plots of land to grow some food to eat, mending their tools and clothes, and going to church if it was allowed. However, they did sometimes shave each other's faces and cut and style each other's hair as much as they could. Sometimes hair was styled once a week for church.

Slave owners often controlled how the enslaved Africans wore their hair, especially those who worked in their homes. Sometimes hair, especially women's, was shaved off as a punishment. This was especially cruel because even though they didn't have much time and didn't usually have combs or hair oils, when they could, the enslaved people styled their hair as a way to express their identity and a have a little bit of personal freedom in their life.

Over time, enslaved Africans began to wear hairstyles that were quite different to the styles worn in Africa. In the 1700s, wigs made from the hair of other Europeans were the fashion, especially for wealthy white men in Britain and in North America.

The picture on page 22 shows Alic, an enslaved personal servant in Virginia in 1797. He wears a plait at the back of his hair like the wigs white men wore but the rest of his hairstyle isn't exactly the same as the European fashion.

RUNNING AWAY

The life of an enslaved person was full of hardship and brutality, so many people tried to escape to freedom. In some colonies, like the smaller British Caribbean islands, it was difficult for the enslaved people to run away. However, in larger colonies like Jamaica and North America they sometimes escaped to places where they could hide and form their own communities. As in Britain, when enslaved people ran away their owners sometimes placed adverts in the newspapers offering a reward to anyone who found and brought them back. These runaway adverts sometimes describe hairstyles, usually men's because it was harder for women to run away. Some enslaved people wore their hair long and unplaited. Some wore hairstyles with neat partings. Others wore hair that was partly shaved.

THE 1800S

From the beginning, Africans resisted their enslavement in many ways. After many years of a growing abolition movement by Africans who had been enslaved and Europeans who also thought that slavery was a great evil, in the 1800s European nations began to abolish their slave trades and then emancipate (set free) their enslaved workers.

The descendants of enslaved Africans had nowhere else to go so they still lived in poor conditions in the same places outside of Africa where their foreparents had been forced to work. Life was still hard. Because they had worked for Europeans for centuries without pay, most people had very little money. Afro haircare as an **industry** didn't exist. Most Black people in the British Caribbean and in America had their hair styled at home by family or friends free of charge.

Women usually wore their hair in simple plaited or **cornrowed** styles. Sometimes they wore a head scarf over their hair. Most men wore their hair cut short. In America in particular, people began seeing advertising which told them that they should buy products to smooth out their coily hair. Sometimes people tried to change their Afro hair using harsh chemicals that could damage the hair and scalp.

THE SCRAMBLE FOR AFRICA

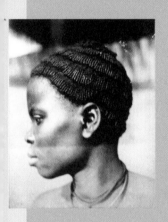

Meanwhile in Africa, in the late 1880s, European nations started a new stage of colonization, known as imperialism. They decided to claim colonies all over the African continent.

European colonizers who went to Africa during this period sometimes took photographs of the traditional hairstyles they saw. These photographs show us that some people in Africa still wore traditional hairstyles in the early 20th century. The photo on page 28 shows an elite woman a hundred years ago in West Africa (today's Nigeria). Her hairstyle is similar to the hairstyle worn by the ancient Egyptian queen, Kawit, four thousand years earlier and Benin elites three hundred years earlier.

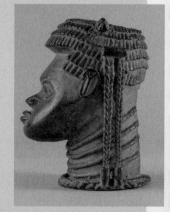

The start of the 20th century saw the birth of the modern Afro hair care industry. It began in the USA and then spread to other parts of the world where people had Afro hair.

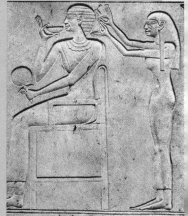

THE BIRTH OF THE MODERN AFRO HAIRCARE INDUSTRY

At the start of the twentieth century France still led the way in fashionable hairstyles for people of European descent in England and America. Men wore their hair cut short (sometimes with a parting). Fashionable white women in Edwardian Britain (1901–1910) wore their hair in a pompadour style. The pompadour was a European hairstyle named after Madame de Pompadour, the girlfriend of a French king, Louis XV. The hairstyle needed long hair piled up and worn high above the forehead.

In the USA, this pompadour style was called the Gibson Girl. Gibson Girl was created by an artist and she appeared in magazines. Gibson Girl had thin lips, a thin nose and pale white skin, but many African American women wanted to look like her too. However, many

African Americans suffered with terrible scalp and hair problems. Life was often still as hard and stressful as during the days of enslavement. As a result, poor living and working conditions made people sick. These illnesses included scalp diseases. People could not afford the best food available, so their diets were poor. And, at that time in rural areas most Americans did not have indoor plumbing in their homes. People of all backgrounds didn't wash their hair as often as we do today.

But two African American women were about to become very wealthy as pioneers of the Afro hair care industry. Their star products were their 'Wonderful Hair Growers' designed to help women with Afro hair grow their hair and heal their scalps.

CHAPTER FIVE: FROM TRAGEDY TO TRIUMPH

In 1918, a 34-room mansion was built on Irving-on-Hudson in New York. This area was where some of America's richest families lived at the time. The new mansion was near the homes of John D. Rockefeller and Jay Gould. They were two white American men who are considered two of the wealthiest Americans in history.

Newspaper reporters and people in the area were very curious: '*Who was building this beautiful home?*' When they found out who would be living there, they were stunned:

"Impossible!"

"No such woman of her race could afford such a place."

The mansion belonged to a Black woman called

Madam C.J. Walker. Her life story began fifty years earlier.

Madam C.J. Walker was born as Sarah Breedlove in Delta, Louisiana in 1867. She was born in a one-room cabin on a plantation where her parents and older brothers and sister had all been enslaved. In fact, Sarah was the first baby in her family who was born free.

Sarah's parents died when she was six years old, and she was raised by her older sister. Life was very hard for the two sisters.

When she grew up Sarah got married. She and her husband, Moses, had a daughter called Lelia. But then Sarah's husband died when little Lelia was two years old. Sarah took little Lelia and moved to St Louis in Missouri where her three older brothers now lived.

Sarah moved to St Louis, a big city, hoping for a better life. But life wasn't easy in St Louis either. There were jobs but the factories were white owned and they preferred to employ white people. Black men and women were expected to do menial jobs.

Sarah worked as a maid at first. Then she became a washerwoman. Sarah worked hard but she was so stressed and worried about the future. Her hair began to fall out because of stress and scalp disease:

"As I bent over the washboard, and looked at my arms buried in soapsuds, I said to myself: "What are you going to do when you grow old and your back gets stiff? Who is going to take care of your little girl?"

Then she met another African American woman called Annie Turnbo Malone. Sarah's life was about to change.

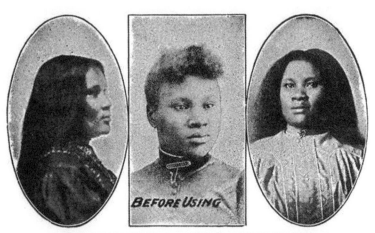
Madam Walker before and after her wonderful discovery.

Like Sarah, Annie had been born free although her parents had once been enslaved too. Annie's parents also died when she was very little. Like Sarah, Annie was raised by an older sister. As a child, Annie loved hair and chemistry. She practised haircare on her sister and her friends. When Annie grew up she went around door to door selling her Wonderful

Hair Grower to African American women. Annie's products were a hit. She decided to move from Lovejoy, Illinois where she lived to the big city of St Louis, Missouri. There were more people there so she would have more customers.

In 1902 Annie moved to St Louis. She decided to give her business a name, Poro. She began training other African American women on how to use her products. They could then go around door to door giving Poro treatments and selling products like Annie's Wonderful Hair Grower. The sales agent could keep some of the money for themselves and give the rest to Annie.

PORO
PRESSING OIL
TO SOFTEN AND OIL
THE STRANDS OF
THE HAIR

One day Annie and Sarah Breedlove met each other. Sarah began working for Annie as one of her Poro sales agents in St Louis. Shortly after, in 1905, Sarah moved to Denver, Colorado. At first she

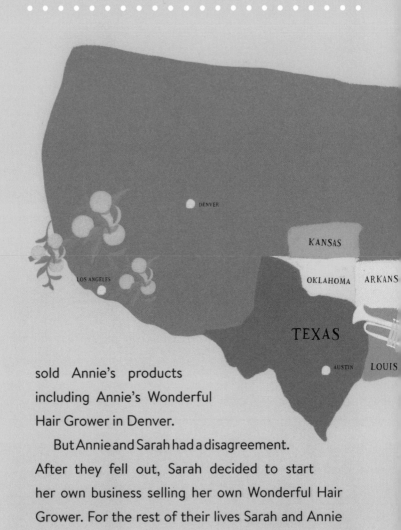

sold Annie's products
including Annie's Wonderful
Hair Grower in Denver.

But Annie and Sarah had a disagreement.
After they fell out, Sarah decided to start
her own business selling her own Wonderful Hair
Grower. For the rest of their lives Sarah and Annie

were fierce rivals.

Sarah had just married a man called Charles Joseph Walker (C.J. for short). She began calling herself Madam C.J. Walker.

Mr C.J. Walker and Madam C.J. Walker travelled around the country for the next year and a half. In those days nearly all African Americans still lived in the South. Mr and Madam C.J. Walker visited many states like Oklahoma, Texas, Kansas, Arkansas, Louisiana, Mississippi and Alabama. Everywhere they went, Madam C.J. Walker gave talks and showed women her Walker system to have healthy scalps and grow their hair. She trained sales agents and took orders for her Wonderful Hair Grower, vegetable shampoo and **pressing oil**.

NEW YORK

TROIT

NEW JERSEY

DIANAPOLIS

ATLANTIC CITY

VIRGINIA

NORTH CAROLINA

SOUTH CAROLINA

ATLANTA

GEORGIA

FLORIDA

NS

MIAMI

They got lots of orders and people said great things about Madam C.J. Walker's Wonderful Hair Grower. One woman who once wore false hair grew so much of her own that she later wrote, 'My hair was the talk of the town.'

In 1910, just four years after starting to sell her own Wonderful Hair Grower, business was so good that Madam built a factory in Indianapolis, Indiana to manufacture her products. She also opened a beauty salon and a beauty school.

But Madam and C.J. weren't getting on well. One of their differences was about the business. C.J. wanted to keep the business small but Madam wanted to do much more. Although he later regretted it, they divorced and Madam C.J. Walker continued to grow her business with the help of her daughter, Lelia.

In 1913, Madam took a two-month trip outside the USA. It was a holiday but she also wanted to expand her business to other countries where people had Afro hair. So she visited Jamaica, which was still a British

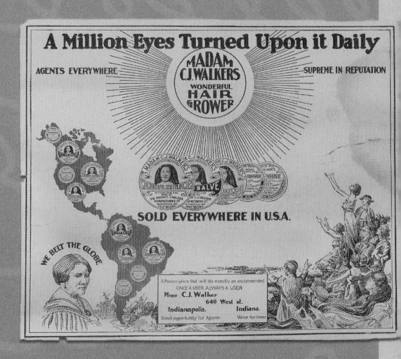

A Million Eyes Turned Upon it Daily

AGENTS EVERYWHERE

MADAM C.J.WALKERS WONDERFUL HAIR GROWER

SUPREME IN REPUTATION

SOLD EVERYWHERE IN U.S.A.

WE BELT THE GLOBE

A Prescription that will do exactly as recommended.
ONCE A USER ALWAYS A USER
Mme C.J. Walker
640 West st.
Indianapolis.   Indiana.
Great opportunity for Agents   Write for terms

colony at the time. She also visited Haiti, Costa Rica, Cuba and the Panama Canal Zone. At the time, many African Caribbean people from Barbados, Jamaica and the other British Caribbean colonies were living and working in the Panama Canal Zone.

Although she worked very hard Madam C.J. Walker enjoyed life. She and Lelia loved giving parties, driving around sightseeing in their fancy car and shopping. At a time when Black women were expected to be domestics, Madam had become a wealthy, elegant and celebrated businesswoman.

Lelia loved Harlem in New York. She told her mother that Harlem was becoming an important place for Black people. So, in 1913 Madam C.J. Walker opened the Walker Beauty School and Salon in Harlem. It was a four-storey townhouse which had a beauty salon and a beauty school named after Lelia. There were also apartments on the upper floor to live. Lelia was in charge. Finally in 1916 Lelia convinced her mother to move permanently to Harlem to live with her.

A couple of years later, Madam built her 34-room mansion in Irving-on-Hudson in New York. It was designed by Vertner Tandy, a leading African American architect of the day. The mansion was called Villa Lewaro. It was named after the first two

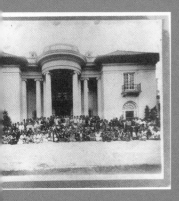

letters of Madam C.J. Walkers's daughter's name: Lelia Walker Robinson.

When she was asked why she wanted a house with so many rooms, Madam replied; 'I want plenty of room in which to entertain my friends. I have worked so hard all of my life that I would like to rest.'

When Madam C.J. Walker died in May 1919 she was at the height of her fame. She had created jobs for others and supported other Black businesses like the African American newspapers where she placed advertisements about her Afro hair products. She gave away a lot of money to charities and inspired many other Black women.

Today she holds the Guinness World Record as the first **self-made** millionairess in the USA.

CHAPTER SIX: THE 1920S

Madam C.J. Walker died in 1919. Her daughter Lelia wasn't as interested in the hair business as her mother had been. She said:

"...People are not as much interested in whether their hair grows or not, due probably to the short hair or bobbed hair style and there are numbers of similar preparations on the market that seem to grow hair as fast as ours."

Lelia was right about both things. Hairstyles *were* changing and there were other good hair products for Afro hair. One of them was Annie Malone's Poro hair products. Annie was still living in St Louis, Missouri. In 1918 she had opened her Poro College.

It was a school to teach Poro haircare and a factory. Annie's business was soaring. Her hair products and beauty salons also reached Harlem.

In the 1920s the fashion for long hair changed so hair growers were no longer in demand. Instead, following the fashion from France, short bobs became the latest must-have hairstyle for stylish women.

In 1922 Lelia changed her first name. She added A' to become A'Lelia. A'Lelia became more involved with the arts. As a rich heiress she had lots of money which she used to help writers, artists and musicians. She held parties at Villa Lewaro and invited Black poets, bankers, writers, actors, singers, painters and others. The money A'Lelia inherited from Madam C.J. Walker's Afro hair care business played an important role in the 'Harlem Renaissance'.

The Harlem Renaissance was a great period in African American history. African Americans from other parts of the USA especially the South came to Harlem. They were joined by many people of

African descent who came from Britain's Caribbean colonies. A few Africans also made their way to Harlem. Other Black people came from non-English-speaking countries like Puerto Rico and Panama. They all joined the African Americans already living in New York. Harlem became the leading Black city in the world. It became the centre for Black art, music, dance, fashion, literature, and politics.

When Madam C.J. Walker was building up her business in the early years (1906–1910) most African Americans still lived in the rural areas in the South. But over the years, more and more left the poverty and racism of the rural areas for city life. Some went to cities in the South. Others escaped the South completely and headed to cities in the north looking for a better life for themselves and their families.

Although cornrows and plaits were ancient African hairstyles, these styles were not valued or seen as fashionable any more. These hairstyles reminded women of the past. And the past meant poverty and enslavement. Moving to the cities, African American women wanted to look modern and stylish. They wanted to wear hairstyles that the rest of society was wearing. Since the wider society was white and followed hairstyles from France where women had European hair type, African American women needed to change their natural hair texture first. Then they could create the fashionable hairstyles.

HARLEM'S HAIR POWER

To get these fashionable hairstyles women with Afro hair had to change the texture of their hair first. The main way to do that was with a **pressing comb** (sometimes called a hot comb). This was a metal comb that was heated on a fire and then combed through the hair to 'iron out' the natural Afro coils. After the hair was 'pressed' straight, it was then curled and waved using a 'Marcel iron'.

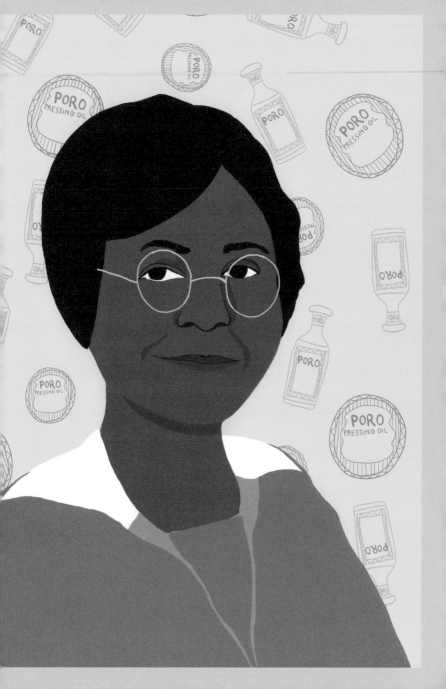

No one knows who invented the pressing comb. The Marcel iron was invented in France in 1872 by Marcel Grateau, who invented the iron to put curls and waves into his customers' European hair type. Marcel later became famous and rich by 'marcelling' the hair of leading French high society women.

Pressing the hair with a hot comb doesn't permanently change Afro hair. Especially if the hair gets wet, the natural coils come back. So women had to regularly have their hair 'pressed'.

The main Black-owned business in Harlem was hair and beauty salons. They did a lot of business 'pressing' and curling their customers' hair. Some men, especially entertainers, sometimes had their hair pressed too.

Afro hairdressers were respected in the community. There was lots of work to do shampooing, pressing and styling hair. Hairdressing gave Black women a choice at a time when it was difficult to get any job apart from cleaning, washing, cooking or other menial jobs. Even if they didn't become wealthy a good hairdresser could earn good money.

According to legend, the first Black-owned beauty shop in New York City was opened in Brooklyn in 1908 by a hairdresser called Madame J. L. Crawford. Madame Crawford had worked as a mobile hairdresser, travelling to her Black and white customers, styling their hair and selling her own handmade products like hair creams, pomades, and wigs.

Later on, in 1911, she opened her second beauty parlour (combined with a dry goods shop). This salon was in Harlem. She had three employees as well as her husband helping to build her business. Then she opened a hat shop with a beauty parlour at the back.

Madame Estelle (Mrs Estelle Hamilton Daniels) was another popular hair stylist and salon owner. She opened the Nu-Life Beauty College in Harlem.

Then in 1913, Madam C.J. Walker who was already well-known in other parts of the country, opened her Walker Beauty School and Salon in Harlem. Her long-time rival Annie Malone also had beauty parlours and a Poro School of Beauty Culture in Harlem.

In 1929, Madame Sara Spencer Washington's Apex System came to Harlem. It became hugely popular.

Soon there were more than 200 beauty shops in Harlem as well as hairdressers who didn't have shops but styled hair from home. These Afro hairdressers all played an important part in making Harlem an important place in Black history. Although most Black women at the time had lowly paid jobs, many of them came to have their hair 'pressed' and styled regularly. They spent their money in hair salons owned by other Black women. These hairdressers, if they did well, employed other Black women (and men) as hairdressers. This helped to build up the Harlem community and support the Harlem Renaissance.

JOSEPHINE BAKER

Josephine Baker was born Freda Josephine McDonald on June 3, 1906 in St Louis, Missouri. Josephine's mother Carrie McDonald worked as a washerwoman in St Louis.

Josephine's childhood was very hard because of poverty and segregation. Segregation meant white people kept Black people away from white people as much as possible. People lived in separate parts of a city, went to different schools, restaurants, hotels, and other places based on their ancestry.

Segregation didn't just mean being separate though. It also meant white people took the better schools, restaurants and other things for themselves. In some parts of the USA segregation was the law.

When she was just eight years old Josephine had to stop going to school. She had to work hard as a maid to earn money for the family.

When she was a teenager Josephine left St Louis behind and joined a group of travelling musicians. Eventually she went to New York and performed with an all-Black cast on Broadway. Next she performed in a show in Harlem.

Then in 1925, when she was nineteen years old, Josephine went to perform in a show in Paris. She became an overnight sensation. Like Britain, France had an empire at the time. Many white French people also had racist colonial attitudes but the country was not as harsh as the USA. Josephine remained in Paris and became a famous star. She became the first Black actor to star in an international movie.

The African American newspapers in the USA reported on all her achievements. The French newspapers followed everything she did commenting on her hair, beauty, style and glamour.

Josephine wore her hair very short in the fashionable bob shape of the 1920s. Sometimes she wore her hair with a parting in the middle and a curl

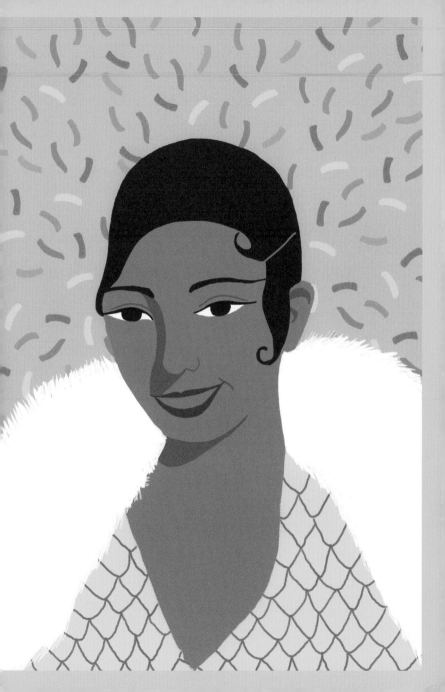

on each cheek. High society white French women wanted her hairstyles. But was it really her hair? Or was she actually bald and the hair was just painted on?

In the 1920s, Vogue magazine told its readers that:

"Her hair, which grows in tight curls, was plastered close to her head and looked as though it were painted on her head with black shellac. The woman is like a living Aubrey Beardsley or Picasso."

Josephine probably straightened her hair with the dangerous 'conk' mixture. Then she slicked it down close to her forehead. Her hairstyle remained glossy and fixed in place no matter how much she sang and danced underneath the hot stage lights.

In the USA from around 1920s many African American men used to 'conk' their hair. Conk was a dangerous home-made mixture of lye and potatoes. Lye is a very dangerous chemical that can damage surfaces. It can burn off the hair and skin.

The mixture would straighten out the coils in Afro hair but it could also damage the hair and burn off the scalp. Women usually pressed their hair regularly but if Afro hair gets wet the natural coils come back. Conked hair stays straight.

Josephine was one of the first celebrities to sell a hair-styling product. It was cleverly called Bakerfix. It was a hair pomade that promised to make the hair shiny and keep it in place without making it greasy. She earned good money from the sales. Bakerfix was so popular that it sold for more than thirty years in the famous French department store called Galeries Lafayette.

CHAPTER SEVEN: THE STORY OF SARA SPENCER WASHINGTON

By the 1930s Apex was one of the most popular Afro haircare brands in the USA. African American hair fashion followed the rest of American society. It was no longer about growing long hair and wearing pompadour styles. Now the fashion was to put curls and waves into the hair. Apex was started by another female African American beauty pioneer. Her name was Sara Spencer Washington.

Sara came to Atlantic City, New Jersey in 1911 from the state of Virginia in the South. Atlantic City in those days was a popular holiday resort for Americans. People came to enjoy the ocean air. Just two years after she arrived, young Sara opened a tiny beauty salon.

In 1919, Sara founded her company called Apex News and Hair Company. Over the next ten years,

Sara built up her business teaching haircare and developing hair and beauty products. She worked in her salon during the day and sold her products door-to-door in the evenings.

She didn't accept that Black people were inferior to white people. She told her employees that they were just as beautiful as anyone else: 'You just have to curl your hair.'

Mary Sadler owned a dress shop in Atlantic City. She remembers Sara well: 'She started a business, and she started the right business.' Sara became a millionaire. A million US dollars was a lot of money in those days!

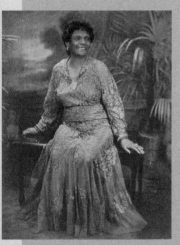

GIVING BACK

In the 1930s Sara used the money she made from her haircare

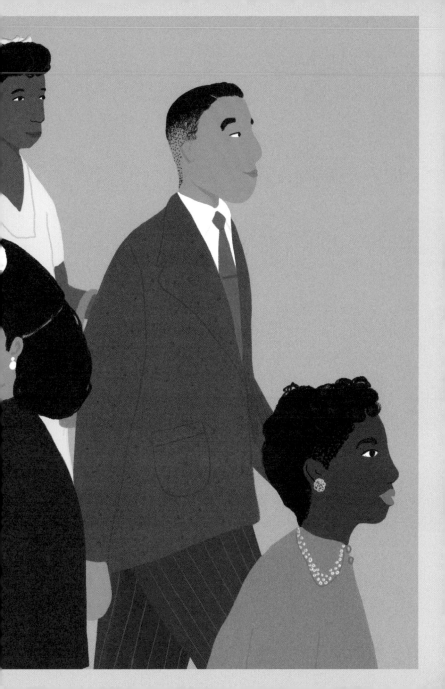

business to buy a **hostelry** that had tennis courts, a dancing pavilion and croquet lawns. She also bought her own farm. The fresh milk, eggs, chicken, fruit and vegetables served in her hostelry came from her own Apex Farm.

Sarah was always generous and gave money to charity. She once gave a party for 1,500 school children in Atlantic City. They had games and a ten-piece orchestra to play music for them. The party food was a chicken dinner, bananas, apples, ice cream, cake and soft drinks.

In 1944, Sarah bought a big hotel called The Brigantine. It was located right on New Jersey's famous Brigantine Beach near Atlantic City.

As well as investing her money in businesses, creating jobs and giving to charity, Sara used her influence and power to help other Black people to enter business and politics.

She helped Black people gain their **civil rights** but she did it through her money and power more

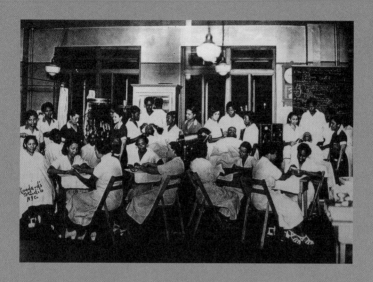

than through protests and marches. In 1945, she famously forced Starn's beachfront seafood restaurant to serve Black customers. When she found out that the white-owned golf clubs in the city weren't allowing Black golfers to enter, she built her own golf club. People of all backgrounds were allowed to play at her Apex Golf Course.

From a small salon Sara built up a hair and beauty empire with 70 different products. She had beauty schools and offices in eleven US cities. Her business was international and she had sales agents in Cuba and Johannesburg in South Africa too.

Like Madam C.J. Walker and Annie Malone before her, Sara Spencer Washington touched many people's lives. These African American female entrepreneurs built up successful businesses selling Afro hair and beauty products. They gave to charities and good causes. They provided jobs for other Black women (and some men too) in their salons, factories and offices. They trained other women who could then look after Afro hair using the Walker, Poro or Apex products. They employed thousands of Black men and women as sales agents. This was a huge achievement at a time when there weren't many opportunities for people of African descent.

Remembering Sara Spencer Washington, Robert Hayes fondly spoke about his days working as an Apex sales agent:

"It was a vision
and a dream to do
something to break
out of that shell where
Black women were just
locked in. And they
had to break out. And
they broke out. And
not only that, they
did something for all
of us. They gave us
a spirit of faith that
there's a possibility."

CHAPTER EIGHT

THE STORY OF DREADLOCKS

In the 1930s a new social and religious **movement** started called Rastafari. Its followers are also called Rastafari. Sometimes they are called Rastafarians (or Rastas for short). The first Rastas were people of African descent living in very poor conditions in Kingston, the capital city of Jamaica. Later on they moved away from Kingston to form their own community at Pinnacle in the hills.

During this time Jamaica was still part of the British empire. The best jobs were kept for white people from Britain or the local white Jamaicans. Rastafari was a protest against this British colonial system in Jamaica. Like the Harlem Renaissance in the USA, Rastafari was also influenced by the teachings of Marcus Mosiah Garvey and an interest in ancient Africa.

Many people in Jamaica did not like the first Rastas. Among other things, they did not like their hairstyle. The earliest Rastas did not wear locks. The hairstyle emerged in the 1950s when Rasta men began to grow their hair into locks. The Rasta men were sometimes called by their hairstyle; first 'locksmen', then 'dreadlocks' or 'natty dread'. Many Jamaicans had never seen this hairstyle, which is now called 'dreadlocks'. In those days, men wore their Afro hair cut short. Long hair on men was considered strange, wild and 'dreadful'. Seeing the Rastas' hair, many people were filled with 'dread' (a very great fear). Sometimes the teachers cut off the Rasta children's dreadlocks when they came to school.

According to one legend, the hairstyle appeared when the early Rastas left Kingston and lived in the Jamaican hills where they didn't have any tools to cut or comb their hair. Their hair became matted and tangled. Another legend says that someone saw a photo of African warriors in a newspaper or magazine and decided to wear the style. Others say wearing dreadlocks became an early part of their religion not to cut or comb their hair (nor for men to shave their beards).

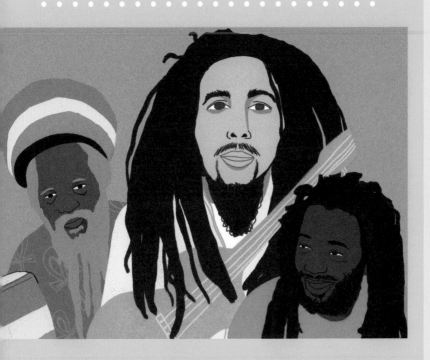

Then, in the early 1970s a popular Jamaican Reggae singer called Robert Nesta 'Bob' Marley became a dreadlocked Rasta. He became the best-known Reggae singer in the world and through him many people learnt about Rastafari. In 1974, Bob Marley and the Wailers released an album called *Natty Dread*. In Jamaica, by this time the word 'dread' symbolized power and freedom. Later it meant 'serious' and 'strict'.

By the 1980s, Caribbean people outside of Jamaica also used the word 'dread' in the same way. A 'dread teacher' meant a strict teacher. Subjects that were hard to learn were called 'dread subjects' and a classmate who was really good at sports was admired as a 'dread athlete'.

Today, some Rastas do use combs and others shave off their beards. Some Rastas do not wear dreadlocks. But for most Rastas wearing a locked hairstyle is an important part of their Rastafari identity.

In the 1980s and early 1990s, some people wanted to wear locked hairstyles but they did not want dreadlocks. So, 'designer locks' became fashionable. See Chapter 15 to find out more.

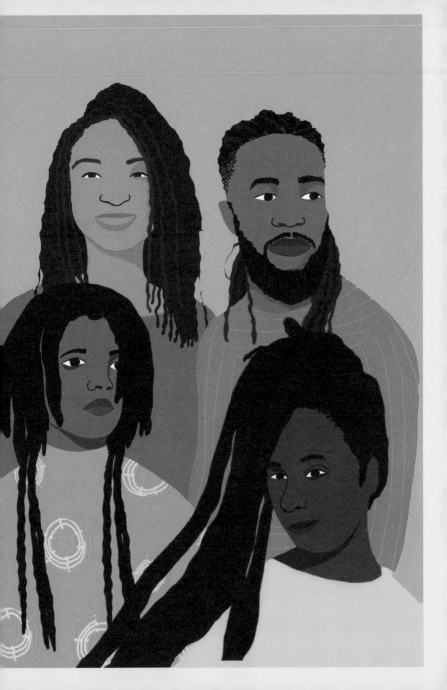

CHAPTER NINE: THE VIOLA DESMOND STORY

he African American beauty pioneers inspired Black women outside the USA too and their products and haircare techniques spread to other places like the Caribbean, South Africa and Canada.

Viola Desmond was a Canadian school teacher. One day Viola read an article about the amazing achievements of Madam C.J. Walker 'and she said, "I want to do that. I want to do that."' So, she decided to follow her dream. Viola gave up teaching and started to study beauty culture. She began learning at home in Canada and then she went to the USA. Viola studied Afro haircare at various places in the USA including Sara Spencer Washington's Apex College of Beauty Culture and Hairdressing in Atlantic City.

When Viola returned to her hometown in Canada, she opened her own beauty salon, Vi's Studio of Beauty Culture. It was a success. A few years later Viola opened the Desmond School of

Beauty Culture to train and help other Black women who wanted to learn Afro haircare and become businesswomen too.

Viola worked very hard to build up her Afro hair and beauty business. She also learnt how to make wigs and she made her own products including a hair pomade. Viola paid her youngest sister, Wanda, fifty cents a week to fill up the hair pomade into the tins.

SITTING DOWN

On 8 November 1946, Viola was driving to deliver products in another town when her car broke down. She found a garage, but the mechanic told Viola it would take a while to fix her car. So, Viola decided to watch a movie while she waited. She went to a cinema called the Roseland Theatre, bought a ticket and went to sit down to watch the film. The movie starred Olivia de Havilland, an actress who Viola really liked.

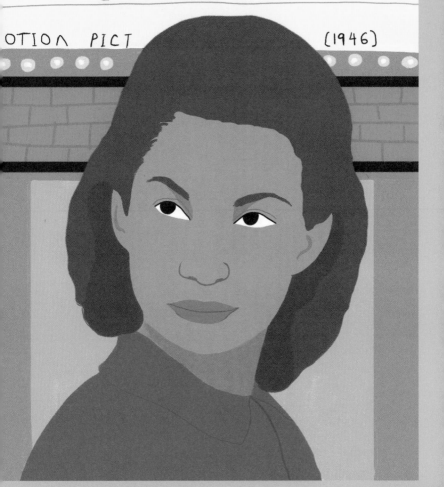

When Viola went to take a seat downstairs, the usher told her that her ticket was for a balcony seat. Viola thought that there was a mistake. So, she went back to the cashier to pay extra for a ticket to sit in the main stalls. The cashier told her:

"I'm not permitted to sell downstairs tickets to you people"

In the Roseland Theatre, only white people were allowed to sit downstairs in the main stalls. Black people had to sit up in the balcony further away from the screen. The Roseland Theatre, like many other places in Canada at the time, could legally refuse people services based on their skin colour.

Viola didn't think it was right that she had to sit in the balcony. She was a successful businesswoman.

She had enough money to pay the small difference in price for a better seat. Viola decided to sit down in a seat in the main stalls anyway. Then the manager came and told Viola to move to the balcony. But Viola refused to give up her seat. The manager called the police who came, arrested Viola and put her in jail overnight.

The next day Viola was charged and found guilty of not paying the proper price for her ticket. She had to pay a $26 fine. Viola had a lot of support from the Black community. They wanted the courts to change their decision and cancel Viola's fine. But the courts refused.

Although Viola didn't win the case and the courts didn't change their decision, her bravery in challenging injustice and unequal treatment inspired the Black community to continue the struggle for human rights and civil rights for Black people in Canada.

CHAPTER TEN: COMING TO BRITAIN: THE WINDRUSH GENERATION

efore the Second World War (1939–1945) Britain did not have as many Afro hair salons as it does today. There have been Black people in Britain for centuries however the numbers greatly increased after the arrival of *HMT Empire Windrush* in 1948. Although Britain had claimed many colonies in Africa and the Caribbean it wasn't common for people to come from those countries in large numbers. At this time most African Caribbean people who wanted to escape from the harsh conditions in the British Caribbean emigrated to the USA.

Before the arrival of the 'Windrush generation', most white British people only saw Black people in movies or in books. When a white British person saw a Black person they sometimes tried to touch their skin or hair. Sometimes people were unkind and didn't show respect. Sometimes teachers and other people even wanted to cut off some Afro hair to take away.

CARMEN ENGLAND'S SALONS

Britain's first-known Afro hair salon was opened in 1948 by Carmen England. Carmen came to Britain from the island colony of Trinidad. She used her 'secret oils' and a pressing comb to make the hair straight and then style it. A 1948 film was made of Carmen in her salon. It explained to British viewers that if the Afro hair 'gets really wet or steamed up, it unstraightens itself and' the natural coils come back.

Carmen's salon was located inside the British Colonies Club in Trafalgar Square in central London. It closed a few years later but in 1955 she opened another salon. The opening was mentioned in the *Daily Mail* newspaper. Readers were told that Carmen was the first specialist to open a hair salon like this in London. The newspaper told its readers that there weren't many places in London at the time where Caribbean and African women could go to get their hair 'straightened out ... and a modern style set in its place.' The article went on to say that Carmen had been trained in hair dressing in Harlem in New York.

Carmen's salon was also a place for Black women to meet each other. It had a social club as well. Another Trinidadian woman called Althea McNish painted the murals for the club. Althea became a famous artist.

CARMEN, CLAUDIA AND THE CARIBBEAN CARNIVAL QUEEN

That same year, in 1955, a woman called Claudia Jones came to Britain. Like Carmen, Claudia was from Trinidad. When Claudia was a little girl in the 1920s, her family moved to Harlem in the USA like so many others from the British Caribbean colonies.

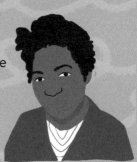

Claudia grew up in Harlem in great poverty.

When she was an adult Claudia began to speak out against racism, colonialism and other types of oppression based on gender and class. She became a communist and was deported from the USA and sent to Britain. As soon as she arrived in Britain, Claudia decided to continue her work against various forms of oppression.

After the 1958 race riots in Notting Hill and Nottingham, Claudia decided to organize a Caribbean carnival. She brought together lots of people from the Black community to help her. The carnival judges included Amy Ashwood Garvey, Cy Grant, Carmen England and many others.

WINIFRED'S SALONS

By this time another Afro hair salon had been opened in London by a glamorous musician called Winifred Atwell. Like Carmen and Claudia, Winifred was born in Trinidad. She loved music and could play the piano from an early age. First, she went to New York to study music and then, in 1945, she came to Britain. She soon got a recording contract and became the first Black musician to sell more than a million records in the UK.

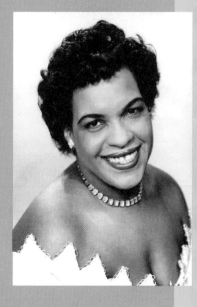

Isabelle Lucas came to London in 1954 from Canada. She came to London to study singing. Isabelle became a singer and an actress:

"I didn't come here from the Caribbean so, on my arrival in this country, I didn't have any black friends or contacts. When I came to Britain and entered 'show business' I had no one to advise me about how to present myself on stage or at auditions. In those days there were no beauty salons for Black women in this country. Black women styled their hair in their kitchens. I needed advice on how to straighten and style my hair, but I didn't know any Black women in Britain. I had only heard of Winifred Atwell..."

Although Isabelle had decided to look for Winifred Atwell's phone number in the London telephone directory, she was a bit surprised to actually find it. Winifred was a big star! Isabelle was even more surprised when Winifred not only answered the phone but also invited Isabelle to her home in Hampstead:

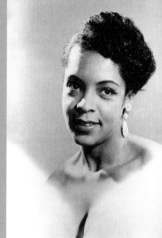

'...Winifred gave me some hair straightening irons. A few years later, in Brixton, she opened one of the first hairdressing and beauty salons for black women. Winifred was so helpful and nice...'

The salon Winifred opened in 1957 was called Directions: John Fior. It was located in Brixton, south London. Huge crowds of white British people gathered outside the salon on the first day. They didn't come to have their hair done. They just wanted to see Winifred.

Winifred was a wealthy celebrity. She had enough money of her own to open her Afro hair salon without going to a bank for a loan. Her salon cost £30,000 which is about half a million pounds in today's money. Winifred also developed an early type of **chemical hair relaxer** called Stay-Straight. However, other Black hair salons had to import their Afro hair products from the USA.

Although her Brixton salon was a success, a few years later Winifred moved her salon to New Bond Street in London's West End. It was near the salon of a famous British hairdresser called Vidal Sassoon. At that time, nearly all of the hairdressers in the West End were white men and their clients were wealthier white women.

PRESSING COMBS

When women of the Windrush generation came

to Britain, many of them knew that they wouldn't find hair salons to help them with their hair, so they brought their pressing combs with them. Mrs. Beryl Gittens came to England in 1952 from the British colony of British Guiana (today's Guyana). Beryl had a cousin, Eric, who had served in the RAF helping Britain during the Second World War. When he heard that she planned to come to England, Eric said;

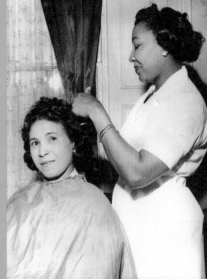

'*Beryl, walk with your pressing comb!*'

Beryl had been a hairdresser in British Guiana. She'd learnt hair care from a renowned hairdresser, Mrs Lucille Dalgetty, who had studied in the USA.

Although Beryl had been a hairdresser before,

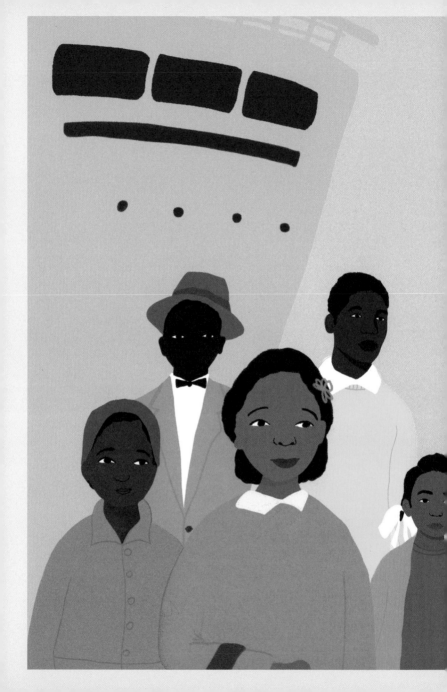

when she arrived in Britain her first job was working in a clothing factory. Some years later, when her children were older, and with the support of her husband Brentnal, Beryl opened a hair salon on Greyhound Lane in Streatham in 1965.

Other Black hairdressers had opened hair salons too. In Birmingham, two small Black-owned hair salons opened in 1960. They were opened by women from the British island colony of Jamaica, Mrs Lyons and Mrs Henry.

Then in the 1970s Winston Isaacs opened Splinters hair salon in London's trendy West End. It was the hair salon of choice for many leading Black men and women. Several of Britain's top Afro hair stylists today were trained by Winston Isaacs.

CHAPTER ELEVEN: THREE MEN CALLED DYKE, DRYDEN & WADE

Although there were now several Black-owned hair salons and barber shops, the Afro hair industry in Britain was still quite small in the 1960s. Most Afro hair care products had to be imported from America. But soon that would change because of three businessmen named Lincoln 'Len' Dyke, Dudley Dryden and Anthony 'Tony' Wade.

Tony Wade came from the Caribbean island colony of Montserrat. When he arrived in Britain in 1954 his first job was 'washing dishes at Lyons Corner House'. It was his first opportunity to make money even though it wasn't what he really wanted to do. Many years later, Tony decided to become a businessman. He set up a trading company called Carib Services.

Len and Dudley were from the island colony of Jamaica. Len believed that Black people should set up their own businesses as a way to overcome unequal treatment and anti-Black racism. He decided

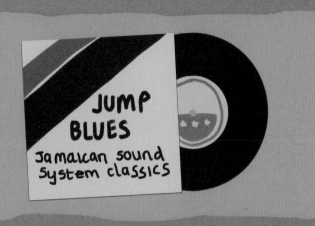

JUMP
BLUES
Jamaican sound
System classics

to set up a music records business. In those days
music was recorded onto round vinyl discs called
records. Len wanted to import records from Jamaica
and sell them to Caribbean music lovers in Britain.

It wasn't easy for Black people in Britain to start
a business in those days. Many British banks didn't
want to lend money to Black people. The white bank
managers denied them business start-up loans.
However, Len's friend Dudley had enough money
of his own to start the business so they became
business partners and started their company in

1965. They named their new company Dyke and Dryden after their last names. They opened a music record shop on West Green Road, Tottenham in north London.

One day, in 1968, Len, Dudley and Tony met and began to talk about their businesses. Len and Dudley invited Tony to join their business. Tony thought about it. He wanted to join them and he knew that three of them together could be successful. But Tony realized that there was another business that could be even better than selling music records.

Tony saw that it was really difficult for Black women in Britain at that time to find the hair products they needed for Afro hair type. Tony wanted to focus on providing 'hair preparations for our ladies'. So Len, Dudley and Tony decided to stop their separate businesses and join together as a team to focus on a totally new business: Afro haircare products for women.

Although the three men owned their new

company equally, they still used the name Dyke and Dryden. Tony didn't add his last name because he thought Dyke, Dryden and Wade was a bit too long. They used Len and Dudley's music record shop in Tottenham for their new business. There wasn't a lot of room as they had to use the space as a shop, office and warehouse to store all the Afro hair and beauty products.

It was hard work building up the business, taking deliveries, carrying boxes and serving customers but the shop was a success. Tony later wrote in one of his books that customers came 'from near and far' to buy their Afro hair products. Soon they opened more shops and warehouses.

Sometimes white people came into the shops. But because they didn't have Afro hair there was nothing for them to buy. Tony thought about their complaints and decided that although Dyke and Dryden would continue to focus mainly on serving Black women who needed Afro hair care and beauty

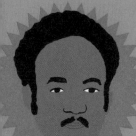

DYKE

DRY DEN

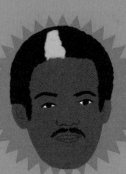

WADE

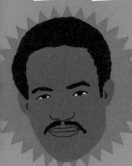

products, they would sell other products too. This meant that they could serve all the customers who wanted to support their business.

As well as shops, Dyke and Dryden decided to help the Afro hair salons in London. So they set up a delivery service to bring the products to them.

At first, Dyke and Dryden imported and sold Afro haircare products from America. Later on, they decided to manufacture them in Britain. This meant business for the white-owned British factories and other companies that made chemical relaxers, shampoos, conditioners, moisturizers, pomades and other products. It also meant business for the white-owned companies that made and delivered items like packaging for the new made-in-Britain Afro hair products.

Even though they were a growing successful business, Dyke and Dryden still faced challenges. Sometimes they didn't get the support from the banks, sometimes they were turned away from opening another shop and sometimes white-owned businesses refused to work with them.

When they decided to manufacture Afro combs in Britain rather than import them from America, it took months to find a company who would work with them.

But by 1987 Dyke and Dryden was on its way to being a multi-million pound business. There were now several shops and they also created an annual Afro Hair & Beauty Show which became a great success.

Len, Dudley and Tony became self-made millionaires and they created jobs for many others. By helping to meet the needs of people with Afro hair, they pioneered Britain's Afro haircare industry and contributed to Britain's economy.

CHAPTER TWELVE: CICELY TYSON

*C*icely Tyson was an African American actress. She was born in Harlem in 1924. Her parents had emigrated to Harlem from the tiny Caribbean island of Nevis. At the time, Nevis was a British colony but, in those days, many African Caribbean people emigrated to the USA, rather than Britain, looking for a better life. In 1962, Cicely shocked audiences when she appeared on TV wearing her short natural hair. Like many Black women in the USA at that time, Cicely usually wore her hair chemically relaxed. However, the day before she was to appear in a Sunday morning drama, Cicely went to Shalimar's barber shop in Harlem. Cicely told the barber to cut her hair as short as possible 'and then I would like to have it shampooed so that it goes back to its natural state'.

In those days Black female stars usually either wore their hair chemically relaxed or they wore wigs. A lot of Black women criticized Cicely for wearing her natural hair on television. But Cicely felt that as an actress it was her job to wear her hair in the style the character she was playing would've worn her hair. Cicely wasn't trying to send a message. She later said: 'Anytime I've changed my hair over the years of my career, it has had nothing to do with me personally.'

Cicely liked wearing her natural Afro hair. She felt 'beautiful with it' and continued to wear it long after the role she was playing had finished.

CICELY'S CORNROWS

In the early 1970s Cicely wore her hair in braided cornrows for a role in a film called *Sounder*. The film was based on a children's book about an African American family who lived in the Deep South during the **Great Depression**. Cicely chose to wear a cornrowed hairstyle because she felt that, 'During the 1930s in the South, poor Black women typically cornrowed their hair, as well as wrapped their heads' while they worked in the fields and kitchens.

Throughout her long life, Cicely was a highly respected actress, an activist and a famous beauty icon known for her elegance and her very different, ever-changing hairstyles: 'Whether you relax it or coil it, weave it or dread it, cover it with a wig or cut it plumb off, the choice is yours. Good hair is your hair – however you decide to wear it.'

Cicely won many of the highest awards for her acting including the Tony, Drama Desk, Outer Critics Circle, three Emmy awards and an honorary Oscar. She has a star on the famous Hollywood Boulevard Walk of Fame.

In 2016, then-US President Barack Obama awarded her the US Presidential Medal of Honor. He said, 'In her long and extraordinary career, Cicely Tyson has not only exceeded as an actor, she has shaped the course of history.'

CHAPTER THIRTEEN: FROM CONKS TO AFROS

(1950S TO 1970S)

he 20th century saw the most dramatic changes in fashionable hairstyles for people of all backgrounds living in Britain and in the USA.

At the start of the 20th century pompadour hairstyles that needed long hair were still in fashion among women of European descent in the USA and in Britain. Later on, fashion conscious women began to cut their hair short especially after the First World War ended in 1918. Throughout the 1920s short bobbed hair was fashionable. Hollywood and European movie stars became the main influencers of fashionable hairstyles from the late 1930s and 40s onwards. Towards the start of the Second World War longer hairstyles became fashionable again. But after the Second World War ended in 1945 the world changed in many ways. As society changed in the 1950s, 60s and 70s, hairstyles changed too.

At first, fashionable Afro hairstyles in the 20th

century were very similar to European hairstyles. However, in the late 1950s stylish people with Afro hair began wearing more hairstyles that showed the natural texture of their hair. Then it became fashionable, especially among younger people, to wear hairstyles that didn't need the hair to be straightened first. One of these hairstyles was even called 'the Afro'.

People with Afro hair have always worn their hair in a natural cut. Sometimes hairstyles from long ago make a comeback. This is because hair type is one of the things that helps to create hairstyles. When a style reappears later on, it usually has a different name. Sometimes it looks slightly different too, especially if other things like culture, religion, climate and leaders have changed.

In the late 1950s and early 1960s short and medium-sized Afros were worn by artists, dancers and musicians like Odetta, Miriam Makeba, Abbey Lincoln and Nina Simone. Cicely Tyson shocked audiences in 1962 when she appeared on TV with

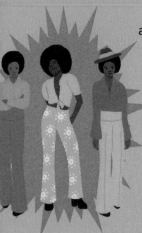

an Afro because at this time Black women were still expected to straighten their hair. Straightened hair was still considered modern and stylish. The pressing comb was still used to straighten the hair but manufactured chemical relaxers were starting to become more common.

At the same time some Black men in the USA, especially entertainers, still wore their hair 'conked'. Their hair was straightened and then sometimes styled with waves. In the 1940s and 50s popular African American entertainers like Nat King Cole and Duke Ellington wore these styles.

As a modern new hairstyle 'the Afro' became popular in the 1960s and 70s during the Civil Rights and Black Power

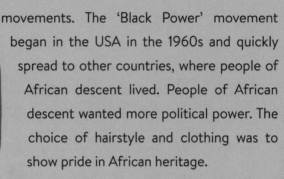

movements. The 'Black Power' movement began in the USA in the 1960s and quickly spread to other countries, where people of African descent lived. People of African descent wanted more political power. The choice of hairstyle and clothing was to show pride in African heritage.

After hundreds of years of often trying to change or cover their natural hair texture, some young people wanted to show that the texture of natural Afro hair is beautiful.

So, they let their hair grow long and combed it with an 'Afro comb'. Many people were shocked by the hairstyle. They just weren't used to seeing natural Afro hair growing up and out into a big round shape. They usually saw Black men with short hair and women with straightened hairstyles. Some people didn't even know that Afro hair type grows up and out rather than down like other hair types.

The hair was grown as long as possible because the style was meant to send a message: 'Black is Beautiful'.

Not everyone was wearing an Afro though. Some trendsetters were following the hairstyles worn by the rest of society. By the 1960s big hair and wigs were also in fashion for people with European hair type.

One of these hairstyles was called the bouffant. Although 'bouffant' sounds like a French word, the hairstyle was invented by a British hairdresser of Italian and French descent called Raymond 'Teasy-Weasy' Bessone. After the Second World War France began to lose its position as the leader in European hairstyles. Instead, Britain started to gain more hair power with its celebrity hairdressers. The African American singers, Diana Ross and the Supremes famously wore the bouffant hairstyle.

A bouffant

Next came another hairstyle invented for European hair type called the beehive. It was even bigger than the bouffant. It was similar to a style that first appeared in Italy in the 1500s. This modern version was named after the place where bees live because of its shape.

When African Americans wore these styles instead of Afros, other Black people sometimes wondered if they were ashamed of their natural Afro hair. Some people did want their hair to be 'straight and shiny' like people with European hair type. However, others just wanted to look like the successful, wealthy African American stars who they saw on TV and in magazines and whom they adored.

WIGS COME BACK AGAIN

Since the end of the 1700s wigs had gone out of fashion among Europeans. But all these bouffants and beehives needed a lot of hair. So wigs came back again.

In the past, when Europeans wore wigs made of real hair, the hair came from other European people. But now there wasn't enough European-type hair available to make the wigs.

Some Hindus shave off their hair and donate it to the Lord Venkateswara. In the past, the priests used to burn the hair but since the 1960s, many temples in India started to collect the hair and sell it. Hair has become a huge export business for India and several other Asian countries.

Not all wigs were made from real human hair though. Wigs were now being made cheaply from synthetic materials.

By the end of the 1970s many people of African descent wanted to wear natural hairstyles. Afros had become more about fashion than politics. Both men and women started to wear cornrowed hairstyles.

CHAPTER FOURTEEN: THE 1980S

In the 1980s, although the internet and mobile phones weren't around yet, most people in Britain had televisions. Hairstyles worn by Black entertainers from the USA were fashionable among people with Afro hair everywhere. The styles travelled around the world when people saw them on TV, in music videos or in magazines and newspapers.

One of these hairstyles was called the Jheri Curl. It was named after a white American chemist and hairdresser of Irish descent called Jheri Redding who many people credit with developing the style. The Jheri Curl used strong-smelling chemicals to first straighten the natural Afro hair and then re-curl it into looser shiny wet-looking curls. To stop the hair becoming dry and damaged from the chemicals, the fashion-conscious wearers needed to use a cream and lots of greasy oil spray every day. The style was worn by both men and women.

A famous African American singer called Michael Jackson wore the style in 1982 for the cover of his *Thriller* album. After Michael Jackson's hair caught fire in 1984 while he was filming a Pepsi advertisement, some furious fans blamed the chemicals in his hairstyle for the accident.

The 1980s saw some of the biggest changes in Afro hairstyles. No longer were Black people mainly choosing to wear styles that were similar to French-influenced European hairstyles as they had since the beginning of the century.

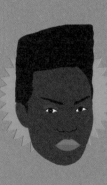

During this decade a hairstyle became fashionable called the High Top Fade. It was a natural hairstyle where the hair was longer on top and very short on the sides and back. Sometimes it was worn with a Flat Top. At the time, it was considered a hairstyle for men and boys. A model, singer and actress called Grace Jones famously broke gender rules when she wore the style. However, a drawing of people from the 1600s shows that women in the kingdom of Benin already wore a very similar high top hairstyle with a flat top hundreds of years earlier.

BLACK BRITISH STYLE

Not all fashionable hairstyles came from the USA. There were now natural African and Black British hairstyles that were in fashion.

Patti Boulaye, an actress, singer, dancer and model, came to England from Nigeria when she was a teenager. In 1978, she appeared on a TV talent show called *New Faces* wearing a long braided hairstyle, which many people in Britain

An example of Funki Dreds

had never seen before. Later on, Patti had her own show on TV called *The Patti Boulaye Show*. Patti's strong make-up and braided hairstyles influenced many Black British women in the 1980s to wear their hair in African-inspired hairstyles.

Then in the late 1980s a group of Black British musical artists called Soul II Soul started a fresh new style called 'Funki Dreds'. Some followers of this 'funky' dreaded hairstyle wore their hair locked in 'dreds' at the top and shaved off around the sides. Others just wore the locks piled up on top of their heads. 'Funki Dreds' was a new way of wearing dreadlocks (which people now often called dreads for short). It was about the clothes and music as well as the hairstyle.

Soul II Soul was formed by Trevor Romeo, a British DJ whose parents came to Britain from the Caribbean island colony of Antigua. Better

known as DJ Jazzie B, when he was older, Jazzie B
explained in a BBC interview:

"During that time of the
80s, it was very important
about our own identity...
We were all heavily into
fashion during that period
of time and then we
created our own hairstyle
... which we called the
'funki dreds'."

Not only had Soul II Soul kicked off a hair fashion
by people with Afro hair, they kicked off a whole
style movement by British people.

CHAPTER FIFTEEN: AFTER THE 1980S

After the 1980s more natural hairstyles became popular. **Box braids** were worn by African American singer and actress Janet Jackson and Jamaican singer Patra.

Then, in the 1990s it became fashionable not to show any natural hair at all. Men often shaved their hair off completely and wore a 'bald look'. Women began wearing **weaves**.

Next came the natural hair movement. More and more people wanted to wear their natural Afro hair. As always, some hairstyles follow the rest of society. People generally were becoming more aware of chemicals in products they bought and used, and of veganism and vegetarianism (which were already a part of the Rastafari culture). People became more aware of plastics and other synthetics ending up in the sea. For other people the natural hair debate was more a political choice. And for others, it's simply fashion. For many people it's a combination of all these things.

FROM DREADLOCKS TO DESIGNER LOCS

Natural Afro hair that is left uncombed will form into locks. The coiler the hair, the quicker locks will form. Various types of locked hairstyles have been worn by different African groups throughout history.

However, Africa is a huge continent. For some groups combing and plaiting the hair was very important so wearing locks or uncombed hairstyles were not part of their culture.

For those groups that wore locks in ancient and medieval Africa the style had very different meanings. In ancient Egypt, Pharaoh Amenemhat III is often shown wearing thick locks. Other ancient Egyptian art shows locks when people are mourning the death of a loved one. In Great Benin, a man wearing locks could be a priest or a bodyguard of the *Oba* (king).

In the 1980s and early 1990s some people of African descent wanted to wear locked hairstyles but they did not want dreadlocks. Dreadlocks are one type of locked hairstyle. Each dreadlock is often a different size or length. The roots of the hair are often not as locked as the rest of the hair.

Instead, 'designer locks' became fashionable. Many people today like to call these 'locs'. These styles look similar to dreadlocks (see the two people at the back of the picture on page 71). However, often these locks are twisted and styled by a skilled stylist. This helps to grow locks that are all the same size, similar length and start from the scalp.

Sometimes the hair is fashioned into hundreds of tiny locks. This style of lots of smaller locks is particularly popular with women and is often called Sisterlocks.

Locks have become a popular hairstyle. Most people with Afro hair who wear locks today are not Rastas. Locked hair is just another natural hairstyle people with Afro hair can easily decide to wear for fashion.

THE NEXT CHAPTER

Today we can see more hairstyles in fashion at the same time like cornrows, plaits, various kinds of twists, puffs, bumps, knots, locks of every possible kind (dreadlocks and other free-forming styles, micro locks, Funki Dreds and more). As well as natural hair of every length, shape and cut, we can see chemically relaxed hair, weaves and wigs too. Even the Jheri Curl look is in fashion again today but without any harsh chemicals.

Like fine art, when we look back at Afro hairstyles throughout the ages, they can tell us a lot about the past. And one day, people will look back at our hairstyles today too. Perhaps they'll say that was a time when people chose hairstyles that showed off the beauty of their faces and their hair.

GLOSSARY

box braids – a plaited style, usually with extensions, where the hair is sectioned into even squares that resemble boxes

chemical relaxer – chemicals applied to the hair to permanently keep the Afro coils straight

civil rights – in the USA, African Americans fought to end legal segregation and obtain certain freedoms and fair treatment under the United States Constitution

clean shaven – without a beard or moustache

colony – a country or geographical area which is ruled by another person, country or government. *See Empire.*

cornrow – a plait made close to the scalp in a straight or curved line. When finished the plait resembles a row of corn or cane. Sometimes also called canerows.

dreadlocks – one type of the many locked hairstyles. In modern times the hairstyle appeared in Jamaica around the 1950s among Rastafarians. *See lock.*

elite – a group of people who are at the top of society

Egyptologist – a scholar who studies the civilization, history and language of ancient Egypt

Empire – a group of lands or colonies under the control of a powerful person, country or government who conquered them. *See Colony.*

Extensions – real or synthetic hair added to the natural hair to add length or thickness

Follicle – a tiny, shaped pocket in the skin which a strand of hair grows out from. The shape of the follicle helps to shape the hair strand.

The Great Depression – a period in world history beginning in 1929 and extending throughout the 1930s that caused great unemployment and worsened poverty. The Depression contributed to anti-colonial protests and the rise of Rastafarianism in Jamaica.

Hostelry – a small hotel that provides food and lodging

Industry – people or companies involved in the same sector of the economy such as travel, music or beauty

Keratin – a protein found in hair, skin and nails. The way the keratin is distributed in the hair strand helps to make Afro hair coily.

Lock – strands of hair left uncombed so that they coil around each other to form a tightly fused unit. Locks can be 'freeform' where the hair has been left uncombed to form into locks (which often vary in size) or 'designer' where the locks are purposely formed to create a specific look. *See dreadlock.*

Movement – a group of people with a shared aim who want to see a certain change or development take place

Olokun – the god of the seas and oceans in Yoruba mythology

Pioneers – people that develop new ways of thinking or doing things

Pressing comb (hot comb) – a metal comb. It was heated on a stove or fire and combed through Afro hair to temporarily iron or press out the natural coils. *See also chemically relaxed and pressing oil.*

Pressing oil – a hairdressing oil applied to the hair before hot combing to help prevent burning and hair damage

Sebum – an oil produced by the sebaceous (oil) gland which coats the skin and hair

Self-made – becoming rich without inheriting or winning one's wealth

Status symbol – a possession that indicates the social position of the owner

Texture – the look and feel of the hair. Afro hair type has many different textures.

Trendsetter – a person who leads in fashion and style

Weave – human or synthetic hair attached directly to the wearer's own hair by sewing or gluing

PHOTO CREDITS

Every effort has been made to ensure that this information is correct at the time of going to print. Any errors will be corrected upon reprint.

Page 10: Limestone relief depicting the queen, Nefertiti © Fitzwilliam Museum, University of Cambridge

Page 16: An Olokun priest. © bpk / Ethnologisches Museum, SMB / Martin Franken.

Page 22: 'Alic, a faithful and humorous old servant belonging to Mr. Bathurst Jones of Hanover'. Courtesy of the Maryland Center for History and Culture, Item ID # RS4717.

Page 28: Photograph by Northcote Thomas, Nigeria, P.119607.NWT ® Museum of Anthropology and Archaeology, University of Cambridge.

Page 29, top: Udo style head, cast in copper alloy. Green, Frederick William, 1950.266 B ® Museum of Anthropology and Archaeology, University of Cambridge.

Page 29, bottom: 'Princess Kawit having her hair dressed, circa 2000BC', https://wellcomecollection.org/works/tyygujhr

Pages 36, 41 and 43: Madam Walker Family Archives/A'Lelia Bundles.

Page 60 and 63: Royston Scott/the estate of Sara Spencer Washington.

Pages 83 and 85: Courtesy of Stephen Bourne.

Page 87: Mrs Beryl Gittens styling hair during her refresher course in the United Kingdom 1958. Courtesy of Sandra Gittens and the Gittens family private collection.

QUOTATION CREDITS

Pages 33, 35, 45: Bundles, A'Lelia, *On Her Own Ground, The Life and Times of Madam C.J. Walker*

Page 56: As quoted in Bryan Hammond and Patrick O'Connor, *Josephine Baker*

Chapter Seven: All quotes are from *The Sara Spencer Washington Story, A Documentary* by Royston Scott

Page 76: Robson, Wanda, *Sister to Courage: Stories from the World of Viola Desmond, Canada's Rosa Parks*

Pages 84 and 85: Bourne, Stephen, *Black in the British Frame, The Black Experience in British Film and Television*

Pages 99 and 100: Tyson, Cicely, *Just As I Am*

Page 115: BBC Four *Soul Britannia* 14 April 2011 clip by Jazzie B on Soul II Soul

FURTHER READING

BOOKS

books marked with an asterix (*) are suitable for younger readers

Ashton, Sally-Ann, *6,000 Years of African Combs* ISBN 9780957443419

Barrett, Sr., Leonard E. *The Rastafarians* ISBN 9780807010273

Bourne, Stephen, *War to Windrush, Black Women in Britain 1939 to 1948* ISBN 9781909762855

Bundles, A'Lelia, *On Her Own Ground, The Life and Times of Madam C.J. Walker* ISBN 9780743431729

*Chimbiri, K.N., *Secrets of the Afro Comb, 6,000 Years of Art and Culture* ISBN 9780956252531

Gittens, Sandra, *Hairdressing for African and Curly Hair Types from a Cross-Cultural Perspective* ISBN 9781861528049

Rowe, Rochelle Rowe, *Imagining Caribbean Womanhood: Race, Nation and Beauty Contests 1929-1970 (Gender in History)*, ISBN 9780719088674

Walker, Robin, Marshall, Vanika, Perry, Paula and Vaughan, Anthony, *Black British History: Black Influences on British Culture (1948 to 2016)* ISBN 9781975619732

Wade, Tony, *The Black Cosmetics Kings* ISBN 9781910553671

ARTICLES

Gill, Tiffany M. 'The First Thing Every Negro Girl Does', *Black Beauty Culture, Racial Politics, and the Construction of Modern Black Womanhood*, 1905-1925

Smith, Kim (2018), 'Honky Tonk Hairdos: Winifred Atwell and the Professionalization of Black Hairdressing in Britain', *Fashion Theory*, 22:6, 593-616

Marika Sherwood's profile of Carmen England in the Black and Asian Studies Newsletter (No. 25) September 1999

INDEX